If you want good results,
you simply must show up,
even when you don't feel
much like showing up.

Dear Reader,

You hold in your hands a fabulous tool for getting and staying fit.

Recording your workouts is key to your fitness success, almost as important as nutrition and recovery.

But this book goes a little beyond the usual data collection system.

Our advancement as humans (along with our experience) is physical, but mental and emotional as well. A good workout journal should almost feel like a scrapbook: it holds snapshots, thoughts, memories, and maybe some chalk marks too. And it's difficult to get that feeling from an app and another backlit screen.

It takes a book: a pen and paper experience with words to drive you onward, focus your thoughts, and pick you up after the world tries to kick you down. A mental workout buddy.

This is what you hold in your hands.

This book is all of what you need in the gym and none of what you don't. If you want workouts or calorie charts or exercise instruction, you can find a myriad of implements online.

This book is you offline. This book is you condensed, undistracted, and vitally fully humanly alive. You and the barbell and the kettlebell and the steel and the iron and the bumpers and the trail and whatever else you use for what is, essentially, active meditation. (Others might call this fitness.)

Read this journal. Savor it, write all over it, draw in it, color in it. Live in these pages. Live so largely that you'll keep this journal and refer back to it, remembering this workout or that failure or that success. Savor all the lessons for they are building you: rep by rep, missed lift by missed lift, PR by PR, moment by moment.

Begin. And, remember: it's never too late to find your beautiful self again.

**With much love,
Lisbeth**

Also by Lisbeth Darsh

Live Like That
Strong Starts In The Mind
Rise
The FUNctional Fitness Coloring & Activity Book for Adults

Strong Starts in the Mind:
Workout Journal #1

Copyright © Lisbeth Darsh 2016

Written and edited by Lisbeth Darsh
Design: Up For Grabs
Cover photography: Tai Randall
All rights reserved

No part of this book may be reproduced in any manner without written permission except in the case of brief quotations included in articles and reviews. For information, please contact Lisbeth Darsh.

ISBN 978-0-9862885-5-5

To contact the author, send email to:
lisbeth.darsh@gmail.com

This journal belongs to:

List 5 goals for the next 150 days:

1.

2.

3.

4.

5.

Now: Cross out two of those goals. Circle the remaining three. Then, focus on those three goals for the next 150 days.

Whatever you face today, put more love into it.

DATE:

NUTRITION: | SLEEP: | SORENESS:
great | *great* | *little bit*
okay | *okay* | *a bunch*
don't ask | *bloody tired* | *holy moly*

WORKOUT:

BRIGHT SPOT TODAY:

Scaling is not an apology or an excuse.

DATE:

NUTRITION: SLEEP: SORENESS:

great great little bit
okay okay a bunch
don't ask bloody tired holy moly

WORKOUT:

BRIGHT SPOT TODAY:

Breathe. Hurt. Suffer. Smile.

DATE:

NUTRITION:
great
okay
don't ask

SLEEP:
great
okay
bloody tired

SORENESS:
little bit
a bunch
holy moly

WORKOUT:

BRIGHT SPOT TODAY:

If you think the weight is heavy, it will feel heavy. Heavy is hard to lift. But light? Light is a cakewalk. You can do light. So tell yourself it's light.

DATE:

NUTRITION:	SLEEP:	SORENESS:
great	*great*	*little bit*
okay	*okay*	*a bunch*
don't ask	*bloody tired*	*holy moly*

WORKOUT:

BRIGHT SPOT TODAY:

THERE WILL COME A DAY.

There will come a day. You will be stronger.
More coordinated. Faster. You will jump higher.
You will lift more. Think more. Love more. Be more.

That day is coming. This day, and all the days
before this one, have been preparation for that day.
You just didn't always see that.

Now you see it. Now you know it. Can plan for it.

Just don't count on it. Because once you accept
anything as a fact, you stop striving for that
anything. You become complacent or lazy or less
edgy. Don't become those things. Don't lose that
edge. Don't become like the others.

Fight to be you. Fight to remain you. But fight
like hell to be a better you.

Remember, the key to all of life is the striving,
the chase, the pursuit of better, faster, stronger
— in body and mind matters. Or matters of the heart.

Striving is key. Pursuit is key. Even if you achieved
something yesterday—anything, even your biggest goal
or dream of all time—well, today is a new day. Don't
sit on your laurels. Throw the laurels to the back
of the room. Look for new laurels.

There will come a day. Keep working towards it.

Tired is all in your mind.

DATE:

NUTRITION:
- great
- okay
- don't ask

SLEEP:
- great
- okay
- bloody tired

SORENESS:
- little bit
- a bunch
- holy moly

WORKOUT:

BRIGHT SPOT TODAY:

> Choose darkness,
> or have faith.
> Of this you can
> be certain:
> Life will reply.

DATE:

NUTRITION:
- great
- okay
- don't ask

SLEEP:
- great
- okay
- bloody tired

SORENESS:
- little bit
- a bunch
- holy moly

WORKOUT:

BRIGHT SPOT TODAY:

> Sometimes, to get to a really good place, you have to go through a really bad time.

DATE:

NUTRITION:	SLEEP:	SORENESS:
great	great	little bit
okay	okay	a bunch
don't ask	bloody tired	holy moly

WORKOUT:

BRIGHT SPOT TODAY:

> If you're going to do something,
> you might as well do it right.

DATE:

NUTRITION:	SLEEP:	SORENESS:
great	great	little bit
okay	okay	a bunch
don't ask	bloody tired	holy moly

WORKOUT:

BRIGHT SPOT TODAY:

Expect more of yourself.

DATE:

NUTRITION:	SLEEP:	SORENESS:
great	*great*	*little bit*
okay	*okay*	*a bunch*
don't ask	*bloody tired*	*holy moly*

WORKOUT:

BRIGHT SPOT TODAY:

Goals are great, but what are the details of your plan to achieve your goals? Have you thought about the details?

Write those details here. Fill all 10 lines, even if one line is "Laugh more" or "Play fetch every week" (with or without a dog). Be specific, but don't make yourself crazy. (This is important in all of life.) Remember: plans are only plans. Real life steps in sometimes. Roll with it. You can follow plans, but you can also change them, adjust them, and throw them away.

But, first, you must make them.

1.

2.

3.

4.

5.

6.

7.

8.

9.

10.

If you want the world to be brighter,
you have to let more light in.

DATE:

NUTRITION:	SLEEP:	SORENESS:
great	great	little bit
okay	okay	a bunch
don't ask	bloody tired	holy moly

WORKOUT:

BRIGHT SPOT TODAY:

> Breathe in, deeply. Hope. And now lift the weight in all of your life.

DATE:

NUTRITION: SLEEP: SORENESS:

great great little bit
okay okay a bunch
don't ask bloody tired holy moly

WORKOUT:

BRIGHT SPOT TODAY:

A woman is never more beautiful than when she is strong.

DATE:

NUTRITION:	SLEEP:	SORENESS:
great	*great*	*little bit*
okay	*okay*	*a bunch*
don't ask	*bloody tired*	*holy moly*

WORKOUT:

BRIGHT SPOT TODAY:

Your workout doesn't make you a better person. What you do with the lessons learned there and the other 23 hours in the day make you a better person.

DATE:

NUTRITION: SLEEP: SORENESS:

great *great* *little bit*

okay *okay* *a bunch*

don't ask *bloody tired* *holy moly*

WORKOUT:

BRIGHT SPOT TODAY:

Don't complain one more day. Only YOU can make it better.

DATE:

NUTRITION:
- great
- okay
- don't ask

SLEEP:
- great
- okay
- bloody tired

SORENESS:
- little bit
- a bunch
- holy moly

WORKOUT:

BRIGHT SPOT TODAY:

If you're brave at the barbell, be brave in all of your life.

DATE:

NUTRITION:	SLEEP:	SORENESS:
great	*great*	*little bit*
okay	*okay*	*a bunch*
don't ask	*bloody tired*	*holy moly*

WORKOUT:

BRIGHT SPOT TODAY:

Sometimes, you have to deal with shit at work and shit at home. Those are the days you feel overwhelmed and you're likely to skip the gym. Don't. Those are the days that save.

DATE:

NUTRITION:	SLEEP:	SORENESS:
great	*great*	*little bit*
okay	*okay*	*a bunch*
don't ask	*bloody tired*	*holy moly*

WORKOUT:

BRIGHT SPOT TODAY:

Hopefully, we're moving beyond broken with every workout and every day.

DATE:

NUTRITION:

great

okay

don't ask

SLEEP:

great

okay

bloody tired

SORENESS:

little bit

a bunch

holy moly

WORKOUT:

BRIGHT SPOT TODAY:

All you have—all you've ever had, really—is heart. A whole lot of heart. Don't give it up now.

DATE:

NUTRITION:	SLEEP:	SORENESS:
great	great	little bit
okay	okay	a bunch
don't ask	bloody tired	holy moly

WORKOUT:

BRIGHT SPOT TODAY:

> It's the rare person who squats too much. Most folks squat too little.

DATE:

NUTRITION: | SLEEP: | SORENESS:
- great
- okay
- don't ask

- great
- okay
- bloody tired

- little bit
- a bunch
- holy moly

WORKOUT:

BRIGHT SPOT TODAY:

A: 5 Things I LOVE Doing in the Gym:

1.

2.

3.

4.

5.

B: 5 Things I DREAD Doing in the Gym:

1.

2.

3.

4.

5.

5 Ways I Could Turn List B into List A:

1.

2.

3.

4.

5.

Doing it badly first is okay. At least you're doing it. Then do it better.

DATE:

NUTRITION:	SLEEP:	SORENESS:
great	great	little bit
okay	okay	a bunch
don't ask	bloody tired	holy moly

WORKOUT:

BRIGHT SPOT TODAY:

What we do when we're injured tells so much. How we fight back—if we fight back—tells a hell of a lot. Don't let yourself be a victim of your own mentality. Fight back and get yourself to whole again.

DATE:

NUTRITION:	SLEEP:	SORENESS:
great	great	little bit
okay	okay	a bunch
don't ask	bloody tired	holy moly

WORKOUT:

BRIGHT SPOT TODAY:

Listen, think, talk. All from the mindset of "What can I learn from this person? How can I help?" Because when you judge people, you lose the opportunity to love them.

DATE:

NUTRITION:	SLEEP:	SORENESS:
great	great	little bit
okay	okay	a bunch
don't ask	bloody tired	holy moly

WORKOUT:

BRIGHT SPOT TODAY:

Step into the rack.
Shoulder your burden.
Breathe.
Your moment is here.
Are you ready?

DATE:

NUTRITION:
- great
- okay
- don't ask

SLEEP:
- great
- okay
- bloody tired

SORENESS:
- little bit
- a bunch
- holy moly

WORKOUT:

BRIGHT SPOT TODAY:

It's not too late to find your beautiful self again.

DATE:

NUTRITION:
- great
- okay
- don't ask

SLEEP:
- great
- okay
- bloody tired

SORENESS:
- little bit
- a bunch
- holy moly

WORKOUT:

BRIGHT SPOT TODAY:

What's in your heart is infinitely more important than what's on your barbell.

DATE:

NUTRITION:	SLEEP:	SORENESS:
great	great	little bit
okay	okay	a bunch
don't ask	bloody tired	holy moly

WORKOUT:

BRIGHT SPOT TODAY:

Keep striving, and don't stop.
We need you to keep going.
You need you to keep going.
Find your excellence.

DATE:

NUTRITION:
- great
- okay
- don't ask

SLEEP:
- great
- okay
- bloody tired

SORENESS:
- little bit
- a bunch
- holy moly

WORKOUT:

BRIGHT SPOT TODAY:

Life is way too short to be miserable.

DATE:

NUTRITION:	SLEEP:	SORENESS:
great	great	little bit
okay	okay	a bunch
don't ask	bloody tired	holy moly

WORKOUT:

BRIGHT SPOT TODAY:

One day, you'll find yourself wondering how you got so lucky, and you'll realize it wasn't luck at all. But right now? Get back to working on your dream.

DATE:

NUTRITION:	SLEEP:	SORENESS:
great	great	little bit
okay	okay	a bunch
don't ask	bloody tired	holy moly

WORKOUT:

BRIGHT SPOT TODAY:

Imagine what your life would be like if you really knew where your red line was. If you knew when to use your power and when to back off, if you knew how much your heart could really take, how much you could suffer, how much you could love, how beautiful you really could be. Imagine if you knew yourself. Now, find out.

DATE:

NUTRITION:	SLEEP:	SORENESS:
great	great	little bit
okay	okay	a bunch
don't ask	bloody tired	holy moly

WORKOUT:

BRIGHT SPOT TODAY:

WORKOUT PLAYLIST.

A.) Name 10 great songs that you would love to hear during your workout.

1.

2.

3.

4.

5.

6.

7.

8.

9.

10.

B.) Make a playlist with those ten songs.

C.) Play those 10 songs in the beginning of your day. Do that for 10 days. Observe how your mood changes. Does it improve or not? Do you have more energy? If so, pick ten more songs and repeat this experiment. Again, assess your results. Figure out what works to put more energy into your life as well as your workout.

Without faith, the bar is always too heavy.

DATE:

NUTRITION:	SLEEP:	SORENESS:
great	great	little bit
okay	okay	a bunch
don't ask	bloody tired	holy moly

WORKOUT:

BRIGHT SPOT TODAY:

Hug somebody. So basic, so simple, and yet so wonderful. Life is worse without hugs, and you know it.

DATE:

NUTRITION:	SLEEP:	SORENESS:
great	great	little bit
okay	okay	a bunch
don't ask	bloody tired	holy moly

WORKOUT:

BRIGHT SPOT TODAY:

EAT THE PAIN.

If the lift was easy, you wouldn't want it.

If the run wasn't hard, you wouldn't race.

If breathing was effortless at this pace, every single person could do it. And then you probably would not want it.

See, easy is easy. Hard takes effort. Achievement takes effort. Success takes effort. Success comes after the pain.

You know that. You probably have success in other areas of your life—you know what elite feels like, you know what winning tastes like, and you love it. As much as you say "I'm competing against myself" there's a person deep down in you who really enjoys beating others. Yeah, you're fighting yourself mostly, but it is a kick to beat someone else. And it's okay to admit it—if not to others, at least to yourself. Be honest, always honest, with yourself.

So, why do you start to fold when it gets really hard? Because there's pain and there's weakness in your mind. Firebreathers do two things in the workout: (1) Minimize their rest, and (2) Go deep into the pain and stay there.

I can teach you how to minimize your rest but I can't teach you how to stay in the pain. You have to will yourself there. You have to learn to live in the darkness for a while. It's not pretty and it's not fun, but it will end. And it will make you a better person, in that workout and hopefully in your life.

Today, put your effort where your mouth is. Swallow hard and bite down on that pain. Bite on your finger, bite on your cheek, do whatever you have to do to get where you want to go in the workout—and maybe in your job and your life.

Bite, chew, and swallow. Eat the pain.

Success is there for the taking. Take it.

So your lift sucks.
Begin again.
So your heart is down.
Begin again.

DATE:

NUTRITION: | SLEEP: | SORENESS:
great | *great* | *little bit*
okay | *okay* | *a bunch*
don't ask | *bloody tired* | *holy moly*

WORKOUT:

BRIGHT SPOT TODAY:

What are you afraid of?
Just admit it, and free yourself.
No one gives your fears
any power but you.

DATE:

NUTRITION:	SLEEP:	SORENESS:
great	great	little bit
okay	okay	a bunch
don't ask	bloody tired	holy moly

WORKOUT:

BRIGHT SPOT TODAY:

Salvation sits right at your feet.
It's just a stupid barbell, but it's one
kick-ass weapon against the darkness.
Against the brutality of the world.
Against the brutality of your own thoughts.
Pick it up and the world gets better,
at least in your own mind.

DATE:

NUTRITION:	SLEEP:	SORENESS:
great	great	little bit
okay	okay	a bunch
don't ask	bloody tired	holy moly

WORKOUT:

BRIGHT SPOT TODAY:

Tired is you vs you. Who will win?

DATE:

NUTRITION:	SLEEP:	SORENESS:
great	great	little bit
okay	okay	a bunch
don't ask	bloody tired	holy moly

WORKOUT:

BRIGHT SPOT TODAY:

When you breathe in, you take so much more than air. You take dreams and love and life and anger and sadness and implacable despair and unconquerable hope. You bring it deep into your lungs, you fill your belly with it all, and then you close your mouth. And you descend with the weight. Whether you rise again is a testament to the strength of you.

DATE:

NUTRITION:	SLEEP:	SORENESS:
great	great	little bit
okay	okay	a bunch
don't ask	bloody tired	holy moly

WORKOUT:

BRIGHT SPOT TODAY:

There's a moment, when you lift the weight from the rack, when you first feel the burden on your back, when you breathe in all that you are about to try, to do, to become. A moment that is somehow small and big at the same time. A moment that determines so much.

DATE:

NUTRITION:	SLEEP:	SORENESS:
great	great	little bit
okay	okay	a bunch
don't ask	bloody tired	holy moly

WORKOUT:

BRIGHT SPOT TODAY:

Be strong now.
In fact, be strong when faced with anything and everything in your life. Tackle it. Do the work.

DATE:

NUTRITION:　　　　　　　SLEEP:　　　　　　　SORENESS:

great　　　　　　　　　great　　　　　　　　little bit

okay　　　　　　　　　　okay　　　　　　　　　a bunch

don't ask　　　　　　　bloody tired　　　　　holy moly

WORKOUT:

BRIGHT SPOT TODAY:

5 amazing things that happened during your training this month:

1.

2.

3.

4.

5.

Savor those moments. Think about how good they felt. When your training isn't going so well, come back to this page and remember. Then, get back to training.

Don't surround yourself with people who demand little of you. Don't fill your life only with people you can easily surpass. Find someone to chase, someone who will help make you better.

DATE:

NUTRITION:	SLEEP:	SORENESS:
great	great	little bit
okay	okay	a bunch
don't ask	bloody tired	holy moly

WORKOUT:

BRIGHT SPOT TODAY:

> The best coaches in this life know when to kick you in the ass and when to hug you. Let them. You're going to be a far better person if you do.

DATE:

NUTRITION:	SLEEP:	SORENESS:
great	great	little bit
okay	okay	a bunch
don't ask	bloody tired	holy moly

WORKOUT:

BRIGHT SPOT TODAY:

They say living well is the best revenge.
Maybe lifting well is the way to get there.

DATE:

NUTRITION:	SLEEP:	SORENESS:
great	great	little bit
okay	okay	a bunch
don't ask	bloody tired	holy moly

WORKOUT:

BRIGHT SPOT TODAY:

The barbell took that angry voice and gave you a new one. And everyone wondered why you sounded so happy. Except those who had met the barbell too.

DATE:

NUTRITION:	SLEEP:	SORENESS:
great	great	little bit
okay	okay	a bunch
don't ask	bloody tired	holy moly

WORKOUT:

BRIGHT SPOT TODAY:

> Every time you tell yourself bullshit, you're limiting yourself.

DATE:

NUTRITION:	SLEEP:	SORENESS:
great	*great*	*little bit*
okay	*okay*	*a bunch*
don't ask	*bloody tired*	*holy moly*

WORKOUT:

BRIGHT SPOT TODAY:

Get to the gym. The road to better doesn't run through your couch or your appointment calendar.
The road to better runs through you.

DATE:

NUTRITION:	SLEEP:	SORENESS:
great	*great*	*little bit*
okay	*okay*	*a bunch*
don't ask	*bloody tired*	*holy moly*

WORKOUT:

BRIGHT SPOT TODAY:

Pain serves its purpose. Life is yelling at you. Listen.

DATE:

NUTRITION:
great
okay
don't ask

SLEEP:
great
okay
bloody tired

SORENESS:
little bit
a bunch
holy moly

WORKOUT:

BRIGHT SPOT TODAY:

One failed lift won't make you a bad person,
a worse parent, a horrible daughter,
an inadequate brother. It was just a weight
that gravity pulled early to Earth,
before you wanted it there.

DATE:

NUTRITION:	SLEEP:	SORENESS:
great	*great*	*little bit*
okay	*okay*	*a bunch*
don't ask	*bloody tired*	*holy moly*

WORKOUT:

BRIGHT SPOT TODAY:

> Be smart. Be courageous. Be bold. Throw everything you've got on the line, and watch life reply.

DATE:

NUTRITION:
- great
- okay
- don't ask

SLEEP:
- great
- okay
- bloody tired

SORENESS:
- little bit
- a bunch
- holy moly

WORKOUT:

BRIGHT SPOT TODAY:

> Sometimes you're going to make it, sometimes you're going to win, sometimes you're going to be smiling and shaking your head at how lucky you are. And sometimes you'll be sitting there feeling like a truck ran you over, wondering what the hell you did wrong. It's all good. Learn.

DATE:

NUTRITION:	SLEEP:	SORENESS:
great	great	little bit
okay	okay	a bunch
don't ask	bloody tired	holy moly

WORKOUT:

BRIGHT SPOT TODAY:

CHECK-IN TIME!

How you're feeling about your goals (circle one):

1. On track! Making progress and feeling great!

2. A little behind. But with some focus, I'll be okay.

3. Way behind. Maybe I should make new goals?

4. What are my goals again?

Now: No matter where you are at this check-in, list three things you can do to stay on track or get on track to goal achievement.

1.

2.

3.

> Once you truly experience the power of the barbell, you can't ever go back.

DATE:

NUTRITION:	SLEEP:	SORENESS:
great	great	little bit
okay	okay	a bunch
don't ask	bloody tired	holy moly

WORKOUT:

BRIGHT SPOT TODAY:

Some linguists maintain that the word "exercise" is derived from the word "exorcise", meaning "to deliver or purify from the influence of an evil spirit or demon." Maybe they're right. Maybe that's what we're doing.

DATE:

NUTRITION:
- great
- okay
- don't ask

SLEEP:
- great
- okay
- bloody tired

SORENESS:
- little bit
- a bunch
- holy moly

WORKOUT:

BRIGHT SPOT TODAY:

Change is born of one person, one mind, one action. Somebody who says "Yeah, this sucks but I'm not going down. Take that, you f***ers!"

DATE:

NUTRITION:	SLEEP:	SORENESS:
great	*great*	*little bit*
okay	*okay*	*a bunch*
don't ask	*bloody tired*	*holy moly*

WORKOUT:

BRIGHT SPOT TODAY:

Don't wait. Do it now. Action is the only way that life is going to get better.

DATE:

NUTRITION: SLEEP: SORENESS:

great   *great*   *little bit*

okay   *okay*   *a bunch*

don't ask   *bloody tired*   *holy moly*

WORKOUT:

BRIGHT SPOT TODAY:

The smart athlete knows when to lift, but the smarter athlete knows when to leave the platform. I'm not saying quit early. I'm saying use your brain and quit at the right time. Be strong in mind as well as body. Sometimes the greater gain awaits you on another day.

DATE:

NUTRITION:	SLEEP:	SORENESS:
great	great	little bit
okay	okay	a bunch
don't ask	bloody tired	holy moly

WORKOUT:

BRIGHT SPOT TODAY:

The world needs you alive. The world needs you vibrant. The world needs you on fire.

DATE:

NUTRITION:	SLEEP:	SORENESS:
great	*great*	*little bit*
okay	*okay*	*a bunch*
don't ask	*bloody tired*	*holy moly*

WORKOUT:

BRIGHT SPOT TODAY:

You're going to mess up a ton of stuff. Lifts will go bad, words will go wrong, mistakes will happen. But don't accept mediocrity. When you fail, try again.

DATE:

NUTRITION:	SLEEP:	SORENESS:
great	great	little bit
okay	okay	a bunch
don't ask	bloody tired	holy moly

WORKOUT:

BRIGHT SPOT TODAY:

Age is not a disability. Stop speaking of it as such.

DATE:

NUTRITION:	SLEEP:	SORENESS:
great	*great*	*little bit*
okay	*okay*	*a bunch*
don't ask	*bloody tired*	*holy moly*

WORKOUT:

BRIGHT SPOT TODAY:

> Gather yourself, address the bar, breathe, and lift. Don't make it more complex in movement or thought than it needs to be. Lift the flippin' bar.

DATE:

NUTRITION:	SLEEP:	SORENESS:
great	great	little bit
okay	okay	a bunch
don't ask	bloody tired	holy moly

WORKOUT:

BRIGHT SPOT TODAY:

Although we might like to imagine otherwise, we are, for the most part, as happy as we choose to be. Happiness is a choice.

DATE:

NUTRITION:	SLEEP:	SORENESS:
great	*great*	*little bit*
okay	*okay*	*a bunch*
don't ask	*bloody tired*	*holy moly*

WORKOUT:

BRIGHT SPOT TODAY:

DREAM WHITEBOARD.

1. Write your dream workout here. Include specifics:
the time you would finish in, the weight you would lift,
or any other salient details.

2. Add your favorite motivational quote.

3. Rip this page out and tape it to your bathroom mirror
until you achieve your goal.

A workout is the perfect opportunity to breathe and move on from whatever sucked in your life today. So, do that.

DATE:

NUTRITION:	SLEEP:	SORENESS:
great	great	little bit
okay	okay	a bunch
don't ask	bloody tired	holy moly

WORKOUT:

BRIGHT SPOT TODAY:

> Working harder is okay, but working smarter is what you really want to do.

DATE:

NUTRITION:	SLEEP:	SORENESS:
great	great	little bit
okay	okay	a bunch
don't ask	bloody tired	holy moly

WORKOUT:

BRIGHT SPOT TODAY:

The world is brutal, and you must be brave. But you have a barbell. You can do something. And then another thing. And another. You change. Things change. We change. Get on it.

DATE:

NUTRITION:	SLEEP:	SORENESS:
great	*great*	*little bit*
okay	*okay*	*a bunch*
don't ask	*bloody tired*	*holy moly*

WORKOUT:

BRIGHT SPOT TODAY:

Don't wait for approval. Go out and be exactly who you want to be.

DATE:

NUTRITION:	SLEEP:	SORENESS:
great	great	little bit
okay	okay	a bunch
don't ask	bloody tired	holy moly

WORKOUT:

BRIGHT SPOT TODAY:

Because there's no point in picking up the bar if you're not ready to lift it. Take time. Get your head right, then approach the bar.

DATE:

NUTRITION:	SLEEP:	SORENESS:
great	*great*	*little bit*
okay	*okay*	*a bunch*
don't ask	*bloody tired*	*holy moly*

WORKOUT:

BRIGHT SPOT TODAY:

Be bold. Be brave. Be big.
And, whenever you can, be kind.
It's way more important than any
of us ever realize.

DATE:

NUTRITION:	SLEEP:	SORENESS:
great	great	little bit
okay	okay	a bunch
don't ask	bloody tired	holy moly

WORKOUT:

BRIGHT SPOT TODAY:

> Firebreathers do two things in the workout: (1) Minimize their rest, and (2) Go deep into the pain and stay there.

DATE: _____

NUTRITION:	SLEEP:	SORENESS:
great	*great*	*little bit*
okay	*okay*	*a bunch*
don't ask	*bloody tired*	*holy moly*

WORKOUT:
_____
_____
_____
_____
_____
_____
_____
_____
_____

BRIGHT SPOT TODAY:
_____
_____

Cheaters think they win.
But everybody knows the truth.

DATE:

NUTRITION:	SLEEP:	SORENESS:
great	great	little bit
okay	okay	a bunch
don't ask	bloody tired	holy moly

WORKOUT:

BRIGHT SPOT TODAY:

Bite, chew, and swallow. Eat the pain. Success is there for the taking. Take it.

DATE:

NUTRITION:
- great
- okay
- don't ask

SLEEP:
- great
- okay
- bloody tired

SORENESS:
- little bit
- a bunch
- holy moly

WORKOUT:

BRIGHT SPOT TODAY:

What you put into life, you get out of life. So don't quit, and don't stop. Drive onward, always onward.

DATE:

NUTRITION:	SLEEP:	SORENESS:
great	great	little bit
okay	okay	a bunch
don't ask	bloody tired	holy moly

WORKOUT:

BRIGHT SPOT TODAY:

1. If you could say one positive thing to yourself every day, it would be this:

2. If you could accomplish one thing at the gym over the next year, it would be this:

3. If you could change one thing about your life, it would be this:

4. If you could have one dream come true, it would be this:

Read all four of your answers. How does your answer to #1 relate to #2, #3, and #4? How do they all relate to each other? Or do they relate at all? What does this tell you? Write it here:

Clean up your attitude. Clean up your words. Clean up your diet. Clean up your relationships. Clean up your life.

DATE:

NUTRITION:	SLEEP:	SORENESS:
great	great	little bit
okay	okay	a bunch
don't ask	bloody tired	holy moly

WORKOUT:

BRIGHT SPOT TODAY:

The barbell is your friend, whether you know it yet or not.

DATE:

NUTRITION:	SLEEP:	SORENESS:
great	great	little bit
okay	okay	a bunch
don't ask	bloody tired	holy moly

WORKOUT:

BRIGHT SPOT TODAY:

Pick the weight up. Throw the weight down. Swear out loud if you want to.

DATE:

NUTRITION:	SLEEP:	SORENESS:
great	great	little bit
okay	okay	a bunch
don't ask	bloody tired	holy moly

WORKOUT:

BRIGHT SPOT TODAY:

Success is reaping the rewards of many difficult moments, each met and conquered. Success is a culmination. But it all starts with the walk through the door.

DATE:

NUTRITION:	SLEEP:	SORENESS:
great	great	little bit
okay	okay	a bunch
don't ask	bloody tired	holy moly

WORKOUT:

BRIGHT SPOT TODAY:

Put on your big girl panties and do the stuff you don't want to do. It's called being a grown-up.

DATE:

NUTRITION:	SLEEP:	SORENESS:
great	*great*	*little bit*
okay	*okay*	*a bunch*
don't ask	*bloody tired*	*holy moly*

WORKOUT:

BRIGHT SPOT TODAY:

Even if you achieved something yesterday—anything, even your biggest goal or dream of all time—well, today is a new day. Don't sit on your laurels. Throw the laurels to the back of the gym. Look for new laurels.

DATE:

NUTRITION:
- great
- okay
- don't ask

SLEEP:
- great
- okay
- bloody tired

SORENESS:
- little bit
- a bunch
- holy moly

WORKOUT:

BRIGHT SPOT TODAY:

DON'T SAVE IT FOR LATER.

Do you save it for later?

Is this your mindset? At least some of the time? In your workout, in your home, in your heart?

"I can't go all out here. Got to save something for later."

"I can't tell her how I feel. Maybe later."

"I should save these old fat pants. I might wear them again one day."

Do you refrigerate food that you know you're never going to eat? Do you keep clothes in your closet that you know you're never going to wear again? Do you hold yourself back (just a little) in the workout because you worry you won't have enough energy at the end? Do you pick a weight on the bar because it's right for you—or because you're scared of what you really could do?

Stop it. Most of the time, you're doing yourself no favors. You'd do better by going a little harder, giving a little more, being more of you. Not all of the time, but most. The stuff you're "saving for later" might actually be weighing you down.

This life is short. No matter how long it seems in any given moment, this life is over in a flash for all of us. So, save when it makes sense, like with money and time. But everything else?

Be smart. Be courageous. Be bold. Throw everything you've got on the line and watch life reply.

Sometimes you're going to make it, sometimes you're going to win, sometimes you're going to be smiling and shaking your head at how lucky you are. And sometimes you'll be sitting there feeling like a truck ran you over, wondering what the hell you did wrong.

It's all good. Just don't save it all for later. Later may never come. But now? Now is waiting for you to kick ass.

I hope you know the thrill of doing one thing with such grace and beauty that it takes your breath away even to think about it.

DATE:

NUTRITION:	SLEEP:	SORENESS:
great	great	little bit
okay	okay	a bunch
don't ask	bloody tired	holy moly

WORKOUT:

BRIGHT SPOT TODAY:

Step up to the bar like you own that thing, not like you're asking permission of it or permission of this life.

DATE:

NUTRITION:	SLEEP:	SORENESS:
great	great	little bit
okay	okay	a bunch
don't ask	bloody tired	holy moly

WORKOUT:

BRIGHT SPOT TODAY:

> What matters is what you do after the wheels are off the bus.

DATE:

NUTRITION:	SLEEP:	SORENESS:
great	great	little bit
okay	okay	a bunch
don't ask	bloody tired	holy moly

WORKOUT:

BRIGHT SPOT TODAY:

3 Things you would like to do in the gym, but have not yet:

1.

2.

3.

3 People who could help you learn/do those things:

1.

2.

3.

Now, ask each one of those people for one tip on how to do that thing you want to do. Write those tips here.

1.

2.

3.

People who don't like deadlifts are like people who don't like dogs: probably not to be trusted.

DATE:

NUTRITION:
- great
- okay
- don't ask

SLEEP:
- great
- okay
- bloody tired

SORENESS:
- little bit
- a bunch
- holy moly

WORKOUT:

BRIGHT SPOT TODAY:

We often have everything we need to start, to change, to become better.

DATE:

NUTRITION:	SLEEP:	SORENESS:
great	great	little bit
okay	okay	a bunch
don't ask	bloody tired	holy moly

WORKOUT:

BRIGHT SPOT TODAY:

Movement is key, even on the days that you don't feel like moving. In fact, movement is more important on those days. Movement is life.

DATE:

NUTRITION:
- great
- okay
- don't ask

SLEEP:
- great
- okay
- bloody tired

SORENESS:
- little bit
- a bunch
- holy moly

WORKOUT:

BRIGHT SPOT TODAY:

What holds most people back is their fear of pain, not the pain itself. It's a mind game, and they lose. Don't be most people. Be stronger—in mind and body.

DATE:

NUTRITION:	SLEEP:	SORENESS:
great	great	little bit
okay	okay	a bunch
don't ask	bloody tired	holy moly

WORKOUT:

BRIGHT SPOT TODAY:

When nothing else seems to work right or be right, the barbell feels right. The barbell makes you feel big, no matter how short or tiny or less-than-powerful you feel. Once that barbell is in your hands, you are 10 feet tall and have an ass that can squat the world.

DATE:

NUTRITION:	SLEEP:	SORENESS:
great	great	little bit
okay	okay	a bunch
don't ask	bloody tired	holy moly

WORKOUT:

BRIGHT SPOT TODAY:

Figure out what you need to do to get strong again. Figure it out and get back to work. Life does not improve unless you improve.

DATE:

NUTRITION:	SLEEP:	SORENESS:
great	*great*	*little bit*
okay	*okay*	*a bunch*
don't ask	*bloody tired*	*holy moly*

WORKOUT:

BRIGHT SPOT TODAY:

The next time you think you're old, take a look at masters athletes, and check your attitude. You are as old as you think you are.

DATE:

NUTRITION:	SLEEP:	SORENESS:
great	*great*	*little bit*
okay	*okay*	*a bunch*
don't ask	*bloody tired*	*holy moly*

WORKOUT:

BRIGHT SPOT TODAY:

I will not go gently into the good night.
I will not let my body spread, my willpower relax,
and my determination downgrade. I am making
a stand here. Like Dylan Thomas, I am raging
against the dying of the light.

DATE:

NUTRITION:	SLEEP:	SORENESS:
great	great	little bit
okay	okay	a bunch
don't ask	bloody tired	holy moly

WORKOUT:

BRIGHT SPOT TODAY:

No matter how bad you feel before the workout, no matter how horrendous your day is until the point that you walk in the gym, you always feel better after the workout. Well, at least once you can breathe again.

DATE:

NUTRITION:	SLEEP:	SORENESS:
great	*great*	*little bit*
okay	*okay*	*a bunch*
don't ask	*bloody tired*	*holy moly*

WORKOUT:

BRIGHT SPOT TODAY:

Most of the time, you're going to do better by going a little harder, giving a little more, being a little bit more of yourself.

DATE:

NUTRITION:	SLEEP:	SORENESS:
great	great	little bit
okay	okay	a bunch
don't ask	bloody tired	holy moly

WORKOUT:

BRIGHT SPOT TODAY:

Success is the result of unyielding, unwavering, and obsessive commitment to the job at hand.

DATE:

NUTRITION:	SLEEP:	SORENESS:
great	great	little bit
okay	okay	a bunch
don't ask	bloody tired	holy moly

WORKOUT:

BRIGHT SPOT TODAY:

We go deeper into the darkness in order to escape, to free ourselves. We go through in order to get through, to emerge in the light, to rise in triumph and exhaustion and gratitude.

DATE:

NUTRITION:	SLEEP:	SORENESS:
great	*great*	*little bit*
okay	*okay*	*a bunch*
don't ask	*bloody tired*	*holy moly*

WORKOUT:

BRIGHT SPOT TODAY:

List 3 people you would love to work out with.
Include the reason(s) why.

1.

2.

3.

Look at your list. Is there any way to achieve any
of these dreams without being a stalker? How could
you do it? List those ways here. Pick one and try.

1.

2.

3.

The unhappiness will always come back until you find a way to make peace with it. So figure out how to make your peace and move forward.

DATE:

NUTRITION:	SLEEP:	SORENESS:
great	great	little bit
okay	okay	a bunch
don't ask	bloody tired	holy moly

WORKOUT:

BRIGHT SPOT TODAY:

Real badasses don't make excuses. They succeed or fail. Then they try again, often at something harder.

DATE:

NUTRITION:	SLEEP:	SORENESS:
great	*great*	*little bit*
okay	*okay*	*a bunch*
don't ask	*bloody tired*	*holy moly*

WORKOUT:

BRIGHT SPOT TODAY:

Don't take what they give you.
You decide what you are worth.

DATE:

NUTRITION:	SLEEP:	SORENESS:
great	great	little bit
okay	okay	a bunch
don't ask	bloody tired	holy moly

WORKOUT:

BRIGHT SPOT TODAY:

> You wouldn't beg for the barbell to be lighter, would you? So why beg for life to be easier?

DATE:

NUTRITION:
- great
- okay
- don't ask

SLEEP:
- great
- okay
- bloody tired

SORENESS:
- little bit
- a bunch
- holy moly

WORKOUT:

BRIGHT SPOT TODAY:

Everyone is tired.
Everyone.
But the successful don't let tired win.
They win instead.

DATE:

NUTRITION:
- great
- okay
- don't ask

SLEEP:
- great
- okay
- bloody tired

SORENESS:
- little bit
- a bunch
- holy moly

WORKOUT:

BRIGHT SPOT TODAY:

> How does love translate to the barbell or the kettlebell or the pull-up bar? Nobody can love thrusters. But maybe, instead of hating and dreading thrusters, you can learn to love what they do for your body, how they make you stronger in body and mind.

DATE:

NUTRITION:	SLEEP:	SORENESS:
great	great	little bit
okay	okay	a bunch
don't ask	bloody tired	holy moly

WORKOUT:

BRIGHT SPOT TODAY:

Don't settle for less.
Don't settle for bullshit.
Don't settle at all.
Fight.

DATE:

NUTRITION:	SLEEP:	SORENESS:
great	great	little bit
okay	okay	a bunch
don't ask	bloody tired	holy moly

WORKOUT:

BRIGHT SPOT TODAY:

Suckage always teaches a lesson.
You just have to train yourself to look for it.
Stop trying to avoid the suck.
The good stuff is on the other side of it.

DATE:

NUTRITION:	SLEEP:	SORENESS:
great	*great*	*little bit*
okay	*okay*	*a bunch*
don't ask	*bloody tired*	*holy moly*

WORKOUT:

BRIGHT SPOT TODAY:

How do you think you are going to get strong? Strong doesn't arrive overnight on your doorstep: some box delivered because you asked for it. Strong is earned. You handle one hard thing after another. That's how you get strong.

DATE:

NUTRITION:	SLEEP:	SORENESS:
great	*great*	*little bit*
okay	*okay*	*a bunch*
don't ask	*bloody tired*	*holy moly*

WORKOUT:

BRIGHT SPOT TODAY:

Work hard in the gym, but remember you can use this time and these ways to become a better person, not just a better athlete.

DATE:

NUTRITION:	SLEEP:	SORENESS:
great	*great*	*little bit*
okay	*okay*	*a bunch*
don't ask	*bloody tired*	*holy moly*

WORKOUT:

BRIGHT SPOT TODAY:

Name 5 things you really enjoy outside the gym:

1.

2.

3.

4.

5.

Now, pick one and go do it. Don't wait until next month. Do it soon. When you're done, come back and write on this page about your adventure.

Stop worrying. Change what you can and press on.
Laugh big. Complain less. Smile/think/love more.
Go hard. Good things will come.

DATE:

NUTRITION:	SLEEP:	SORENESS:
great	*great*	*little bit*
okay	*okay*	*a bunch*
don't ask	*bloody tired*	*holy moly*

WORKOUT:

BRIGHT SPOT TODAY:

You are alive.
Do something with this day.
Don't complain it away.
Live it.

DATE:

NUTRITION:	SLEEP:	SORENESS:
great	*great*	*little bit*
okay	*okay*	*a bunch*
don't ask	*bloody tired*	*holy moly*

WORKOUT:

BRIGHT SPOT TODAY:

Going heavier just means you went heavier, and, depending on the workout, that actually might be the wrong thing to do, especially if it negatively affects your intensity.

DATE:

NUTRITION:	SLEEP:	SORENESS:
great	*great*	*little bit*
okay	*okay*	*a bunch*
don't ask	*bloody tired*	*holy moly*

WORKOUT:

BRIGHT SPOT TODAY:

Your body and your mind tell you to stop, to quit, to take a break. Yet you keep going. Congratulations, you're a survivor. Carry that over into all of your life and you've got a chance at being a success.

DATE:

NUTRITION:	SLEEP:	SORENESS:
great	*great*	*little bit*
okay	*okay*	*a bunch*
don't ask	*bloody tired*	*holy moly*

WORKOUT:

BRIGHT SPOT TODAY:

Never beg for anything. Stand up. Learn to be strong. And take what comes.

DATE:

NUTRITION:	SLEEP:	SORENESS:
great	great	little bit
okay	okay	a bunch
don't ask	bloody tired	holy moly

WORKOUT:

BRIGHT SPOT TODAY:

Action is scary. The weight on the bar is scary. The height of the rope climb is scary. Showing your heart is frightening. But it's all worth it.

DATE:

NUTRITION:	SLEEP:	SORENESS:
great	*great*	*little bit*
okay	*okay*	*a bunch*
don't ask	*bloody tired*	*holy moly*

WORKOUT:

BRIGHT SPOT TODAY:

You can <u>do</u> better.

DATE:

NUTRITION:	SLEEP:	SORENESS:
great	great	little bit
okay	okay	a bunch
don't ask	bloody tired	holy moly

WORKOUT:

BRIGHT SPOT TODAY:

Change your own expectations of what you can deliver, of what you can do, of what you can be. But you can't do that with easy. You can do it with hard.

DATE:

NUTRITION:	SLEEP:	SORENESS:
great	great	little bit
okay	okay	a bunch
don't ask	bloody tired	holy moly

WORKOUT:

BRIGHT SPOT TODAY:

Every situation can seem to suck, or every situation can seem to hold the seeds for growth. Choose well, my friends. And, remember, that happiness is not given, but chosen.

DATE:

NUTRITION:	SLEEP:	SORENESS:
great	*great*	*little bit*
okay	*okay*	*a bunch*
don't ask	*bloody tired*	*holy moly*

WORKOUT:

BRIGHT SPOT TODAY:

Great work—good work—lousy work—no work. Wherever you are in this line, keep moving.

DATE:

NUTRITION:	SLEEP:	SORENESS:
great	great	little bit
okay	okay	a bunch
don't ask	bloody tired	holy moly

WORKOUT:

BRIGHT SPOT TODAY:

There's a better life.
A better way. A better you.
But you have to stand up
and grab your chance.

DATE:

NUTRITION: SLEEP: SORENESS:

great   *great*   *little bit*

okay   *okay*   *a bunch*

don't ask   *bloody tired* *holy moly*

WORKOUT:

BRIGHT SPOT TODAY:

You have to get off your ass every day and work hard for whatever it is that you want. You might get it, you might not, but, if you do it right, the whole trip will be a hell of a lot of fun. Success will be the bonus.

DATE:

NUTRITION:	SLEEP:	SORENESS:
great	great	little bit
okay	okay	a bunch
don't ask	bloody tired	holy moly

WORKOUT:

BRIGHT SPOT TODAY:

IT'S THAT TIME AGAIN! CHECK-IN!

How you're feeling about your goals:

1. On track! Making progress and feeling great!

2. A little behind. But with some focus, I'll be okay.

3. Way behind. Maybe I should make new goals?

4. What are my goals again?

Now: No matter where you are at this check-in, list three things you can do to stay on track or get on track to goal achievement.

1.

2.

3.

Lasting success is the result of hard work. Period. Dot.

DATE:

NUTRITION:	SLEEP:	SORENESS:
great	*great*	*little bit*
okay	*okay*	*a bunch*
don't ask	*bloody tired*	*holy moly*

WORKOUT:

BRIGHT SPOT TODAY:

Pick up the barbell and become who you always wanted to be but were scared to become.

DATE:

NUTRITION:	SLEEP:	SORENESS:
great	great	little bit
okay	okay	a bunch
don't ask	bloody tired	holy moly

WORKOUT:

BRIGHT SPOT TODAY:

Easy is easy. Hard takes effort.
Achievement takes effort.
Success takes effort.
Success comes after the pain.

DATE:

NUTRITION:	SLEEP:	SORENESS:
great	*great*	*little bit*
okay	*okay*	*a bunch*
don't ask	*bloody tired*	*holy moly*

WORKOUT:

BRIGHT SPOT TODAY:

If you could use a few moments of your day to help lift another person, wouldn't that be awesome for both of you?

DATE:

NUTRITION:	SLEEP:	SORENESS:
great	*great*	*little bit*
okay	*okay*	*a bunch*
don't ask	*bloody tired*	*holy moly*

WORKOUT:

BRIGHT SPOT TODAY:

We believe in more weight on the bar, more depth to your squat, less ice in your whiskey, and more love in your heart.

DATE:

NUTRITION:	SLEEP:	SORENESS:
great	great	little bit
okay	okay	a bunch
don't ask	bloody tired	holy moly

WORKOUT:

BRIGHT SPOT TODAY:

> The barbell doesn't care what you look like or what size pants you wear. The barbell cares what you can do.

DATE:

NUTRITION:	SLEEP:	SORENESS:
great	*great*	*little bit*
okay	*okay*	*a bunch*
don't ask	*bloody tired*	*holy moly*

WORKOUT:

BRIGHT SPOT TODAY:

> If you want something, go get it. But don't think it will come overnight. It never does. Be prepared to work hard for years.

DATE:

NUTRITION:	SLEEP:	SORENESS:
great	great	little bit
okay	okay	a bunch
don't ask	bloody tired	holy moly

WORKOUT:

BRIGHT SPOT TODAY:

We get the pain. We've lived the pain. We don't expect it to go away, ever. And we know how to deal with it. We prescribe power cleans for broken hearts.

DATE:

NUTRITION:	SLEEP:	SORENESS:
great	great	little bit
okay	okay	a bunch
don't ask	bloody tired	holy moly

WORKOUT:

BRIGHT SPOT TODAY:

Don't become like the others.
Fight to be you. Fight to remain you.
But fight like hell to be a better you.

DATE:

NUTRITION:	SLEEP:	SORENESS:
great	*great*	*little bit*
okay	*okay*	*a bunch*
don't ask	*bloody tired*	*holy moly*

WORKOUT:

BRIGHT SPOT TODAY:

The simple fact of the matter is that you do not suck as much as you think you do. You can do this. You are doing this.

DATE:

NUTRITION:	SLEEP:	SORENESS:
great	great	little bit
okay	okay	a bunch
don't ask	bloody tired	holy moly

WORKOUT:

BRIGHT SPOT TODAY:

Stop making excuses. Stop explaining failure. Stop looking to take the heat off. What's the worst that happens? You fail. SO WHAT? At least you had a go at it. At least you had guts. At least you showed your big and beautiful heart.

DATE:

NUTRITION:	SLEEP:	SORENESS:
great	*great*	*little bit*
okay	*okay*	*a bunch*
don't ask	*bloody tired*	*holy moly*

WORKOUT:

BRIGHT SPOT TODAY:

Remind me of the better me,
the stronger me, the smarter me.
The one who knows that even on the
days when I only open my eyes
and breathe, I am enough.

DATE:

NUTRITION:	SLEEP:	SORENESS:
great	*great*	*little bit*
okay	*okay*	*a bunch*
don't ask	*bloody tired*	*holy moly*

WORKOUT:

BRIGHT SPOT TODAY:

DRAW A PICTURE OF YOU AT THE GYM ...

Think of yourself as strong, and think of yourself as someone far greater than who you already are.

DATE:

NUTRITION:	SLEEP:	SORENESS:
great	*great*	*little bit*
okay	*okay*	*a bunch*
don't ask	*bloody tired*	*holy moly*

WORKOUT:

BRIGHT SPOT TODAY:

This life is made up of people who take risks, get real, get vulnerable, throw their hearts on the table, kick ass, persevere and just plain rock, and it's made up of people who complain and do nothing. The only thing you really have to figure out is which group you're in, and whether you want to stay there.

DATE:

NUTRITION:	SLEEP:	SORENESS:
great	*great*	*little bit*
okay	*okay*	*a bunch*
don't ask	*bloody tired*	*holy moly*

WORKOUT:

BRIGHT SPOT TODAY:

You can beat me. But not defeat me.
I will dial myself in. I will focus.

DATE:

NUTRITION: SLEEP: SORENESS:

great   *great*   *little bit*

okay   *okay*   *a bunch*

don't ask   *bloody tired*   *holy moly*

WORKOUT:

BRIGHT SPOT TODAY:

PERFECTION IS NOT REALITY.

Stop the madness. You cannot eat perfectly, work out perfectly, live perfectly. Or if you did, you'd be a miserable SOB that no one would ever want to talk to, or work with, or sweat near.

You're going to make mistakes. You're going to screw up. You're going to fall horribly off the wagon sometimes. Derail. In the ditch. Wheels off the bus.

It happens. And it really doesn't matter. What matters is what you do after the wheels are off the bus. Do you pick yourself up and carry on? Or do you go back to your couch and feel sorry for yourself and give up? Or do you try again, but keep making the same mistakes over and over? That's where you really tell me something about yourself and your character.

I'm not interested in the person who never made a mistake. And I'm not interested in the person who made a lot of mistakes and did not learn from them. But I'm really interested in the person who made a lot of mistakes and learned from them and got better. That's the person who can teach us something. That's the person to keep your eyes on. That's the person to stand near and feed off their energy—because that person is going somewhere we want to go.

Someone said this to me: "The stress from pursuing perfection will a lot of times outweigh the benefits." And he's right. Sometimes, we make our own kind of crazy and it's counterproductive to our goals. We think we have to live at 100%, when instead sometimes we'll be at 103%, sometimes at 80%, sometimes at 90%. What matters is your batting average, not each swing of the bat.

So, dial everything in and go like hell, but don't think everything has to be perfect all the time. It can't be. And that's okay. You're going to learn a hell of a lot more from driving that bus with three wheels than you ever did with four. And when you take it into the guardrail (and you will), get out and put the spare on and keep going.

Stop saying "sorry" in this life when you have nothing to be sorry for.

DATE:

NUTRITION:	SLEEP:	SORENESS:
great	great	little bit
okay	okay	a bunch
don't ask	bloody tired	holy moly

WORKOUT:

BRIGHT SPOT TODAY:

> Go get strong, and earn what you so desire. Be glad that you have opportunities to become strong. This is where you are made.

DATE:

NUTRITION:	SLEEP:	SORENESS:
great	*great*	*little bit*
okay	*okay*	*a bunch*
don't ask	*bloody tired*	*holy moly*

WORKOUT:

BRIGHT SPOT TODAY:

Success in one path (or many paths) is not easy. It's not enough to have a gift or a talent or a skill set. Not enough to have drive, persistence, and dedication. You need to bring it all, and you need to bring it at the right time.

DATE:

NUTRITION:	SLEEP:	SORENESS:
great	*great*	*little bit*
okay	*okay*	*a bunch*
don't ask	*bloody tired*	*holy moly*

WORKOUT:

BRIGHT SPOT TODAY:

Bruises are visible memories. Here, you missed. There, you could have done better. Scars teach lessons. Sad lessons maybe, but useful if we are smart. Don't just hurt. Learn.

DATE:

NUTRITION:	SLEEP:	SORENESS:
great	*great*	*little bit*
okay	*okay*	*a bunch*
don't ask	*bloody tired*	*holy moly*

WORKOUT:

BRIGHT SPOT TODAY:

> She could take madness.
> But she was not certain she
> could survive being just
> like everyone else.

DATE:

NUTRITION:	SLEEP:	SORENESS:
great	great	little bit
okay	okay	a bunch
don't ask	bloody tired	holy moly

WORKOUT:

BRIGHT SPOT TODAY:

Remember, as always, you've got two choices:
Quit or persevere.
How you choose determines your future.
Any workout is just practice for your life.
Choose wisely.

DATE:

NUTRITION:	SLEEP:	SORENESS:
great	*great*	*little bit*
okay	*okay*	*a bunch*
don't ask	*bloody tired*	*holy moly*

WORKOUT:

BRIGHT SPOT TODAY:

Stop complaining and dreaming about change. ACT.

DATE:

NUTRITION:	SLEEP:	SORENESS:
great	great	little bit
okay	okay	a bunch
don't ask	bloody tired	holy moly

WORKOUT:

BRIGHT SPOT TODAY:

> Rage on. Don't just live. Rage. The light only dies if you let it. Don't let it. Fight.

DATE:

NUTRITION:	SLEEP:	SORENESS:
great	*great*	*little bit*
okay	*okay*	*a bunch*
don't ask	*bloody tired*	*holy moly*

WORKOUT:

BRIGHT SPOT TODAY:

Stop telling yourself what you are not, and start telling yourself what you could be. Then (and this part is key): work like hell to become that.

DATE:

NUTRITION:	SLEEP:	SORENESS:
great	*great*	*little bit*
okay	*okay*	*a bunch*
don't ask	*bloody tired*	*holy moly*

WORKOUT:

BRIGHT SPOT TODAY:

Remember: The world will paint you into as small of a box as you allow. Don't let the world do that. Decide what your world looks like, how big it is, and how you want to live in it.

DATE:

NUTRITION:	SLEEP:	SORENESS:
great	great	little bit
okay	okay	a bunch
don't ask	bloody tired	holy moly

WORKOUT:

BRIGHT SPOT TODAY:

COLOR THIS PAGE!

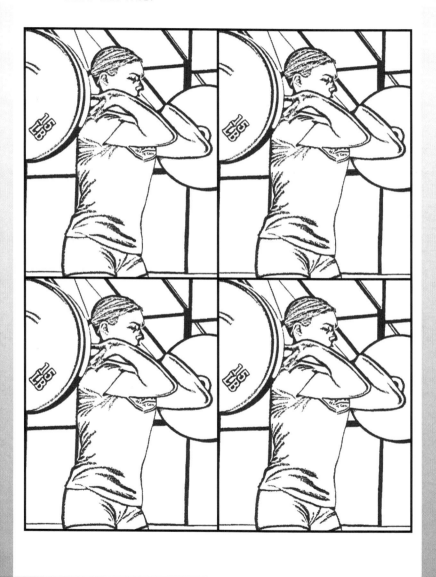

Consider what the pain might be teaching you. Listen to your hurt, and figure out how it can make you better instead of bitter.

DATE:

NUTRITION:	SLEEP:	SORENESS:
great	*great*	*little bit*
okay	*okay*	*a bunch*
don't ask	*bloody tired*	*holy moly*

WORKOUT:

BRIGHT SPOT TODAY:

Whether your life is a flaming success or a burnt-out failure, it all comes down to you.

DATE:

NUTRITION:
- great
- okay
- don't ask

SLEEP:
- great
- okay
- bloody tired

SORENESS:
- little bit
- a bunch
- holy moly

WORKOUT:

BRIGHT SPOT TODAY:

When opportunity presents itself, don't just grab it. Knock it down, toss it on your back, and sprint until you're ready to throw up.

DATE:

NUTRITION:	SLEEP:	SORENESS:
great	*great*	*little bit*
okay	*okay*	*a bunch*
don't ask	*bloody tired*	*holy moly*

WORKOUT:

BRIGHT SPOT TODAY:

Refuse to be defeated. Refuse to go down. Refuse to be one of the ones who never really made it, who never really got what they wanted, who lived a life less than they could have. Fight until your last moment, your last thought, your last breath.

DATE:		
NUTRITION:	SLEEP:	SORENESS:
great	*great*	*little bit*
okay	*okay*	*a bunch*
don't ask	*bloody tired*	*holy moly*

WORKOUT:

BRIGHT SPOT TODAY:

I'm alive and I can feel this life. I'm not anesthetized. I'm not numb. I am here. And I'm breathing. Bring on the challenges. I'm ready.

DATE:

NUTRITION:	SLEEP:	SORENESS:
great	*great*	*little bit*
okay	*okay*	*a bunch*
don't ask	*bloody tired*	*holy moly*

WORKOUT:

BRIGHT SPOT TODAY:

Do your workout today. Go hard, go heavy, go fast. But hug those you love, and keep your priorities in line. Because this life changes in a moment.

DATE:

NUTRITION:	SLEEP:	SORENESS:
great	great	little bit
okay	okay	a bunch
don't ask	bloody tired	holy moly

WORKOUT:

BRIGHT SPOT TODAY:

I will breathe deep and take this burden from the ground to my shoulders, and then over my head. But I will put it down and walk away from it. It does not own me.

DATE:

NUTRITION:	SLEEP:	SORENESS:
great	*great*	*little bit*
okay	*okay*	*a bunch*
don't ask	*bloody tired*	*holy moly*

WORKOUT:

BRIGHT SPOT TODAY:

Be careful, very careful, of the company you keep. These people are also helping to determine your destiny.

DATE: _____

NUTRITION:	SLEEP:	SORENESS:
great	*great*	*little bit*
okay	*okay*	*a bunch*
don't ask	*bloody tired*	*holy moly*

WORKOUT:

BRIGHT SPOT TODAY:

I am not too old for anything. I'm too young for life on the couch.

DATE:

NUTRITION:
- great
- okay
- don't ask

SLEEP:
- great
- okay
- bloody tired

SORENESS:
- little bit
- a bunch
- holy moly

WORKOUT:

BRIGHT SPOT TODAY:

Don't let this world get the best of you. Don't let it take you alive. Don't let this world beat you until you give up. No matter what happens, you keep going.

DATE:

NUTRITION:
great
okay
don't ask

SLEEP:
great
okay
bloody tired

SORENESS:
little bit
a bunch
holy moly

WORKOUT:

BRIGHT SPOT TODAY:

Make no mistake, you can never defeat me. It's simply not possible. I am unstoppable.

DATE:

NUTRITION:
great
okay
don't ask

SLEEP:
great
okay
bloody tired

SORENESS:
little bit
a bunch
holy moly

WORKOUT:

BRIGHT SPOT TODAY:

If you're somewhere in life where the vague ghosts of discontent flutter in your stomach daily and haunt your dreams at night, take heart. You are alive. There is hope. Work, and find your way.

DATE:

NUTRITION:	SLEEP:	SORENESS:
great	great	little bit
okay	okay	a bunch
don't ask	bloody tired	holy moly

WORKOUT:

BRIGHT SPOT TODAY:

You can live the rest of your days as less than you could be. Or you can do the work and become more than you ever dreamed possible.

DATE:

NUTRITION:	SLEEP:	SORENESS:
great	*great*	*little bit*
okay	*okay*	*a bunch*
don't ask	*bloody tired*	*holy moly*

WORKOUT:

BRIGHT SPOT TODAY:

UNSTOPPABLE.

You can beat me. But not defeat me.

I will dial myself in. I will focus.

You can run faster than me. But you cannot run truer.

I will learn to sprint. And to slow my pace for recovery.

You can post greater numbers on every whiteboard that exists in this world, but your weights only mean something to you, not to me. I am my own yardstick.

I will breathe deep and take this burden from the ground to my shoulders, and then over my head. But I will put it down and walk away from it. It does not own me.

Although we pen our efforts for everyone to see, I was never competing with you to begin with. I am trying to be a better version of me, every single workout and every single day. You only help me to get there. Thank you. I hope my efforts drive you harder too.

But make no mistake, you can never defeat me.

It's simply not possible.

I am unstoppable.

Seize this day like no other that went before it. Like no other that could ever come after it. Because you only have this day, or rather maybe this hour, but really only this minute. Right here. Right now. Breathe. Act.

DATE:

NUTRITION:	SLEEP:	SORENESS:
great	*great*	*little bit*
okay	*okay*	*a bunch*
don't ask	*bloody tired*	*holy moly*

WORKOUT:

BRIGHT SPOT TODAY:

PROGRESS ASSESSMENT.

You started this journey 150 entries ago.
Think and answer:

1. Are you in better physical shape since you started?
Yes / No

2. Are you in better mental shape since you started?
Yes / No

3. If either of your answers were "no" what can you do now to help yourself?

4. Go back to Page 1 of this book. Look at your goals. Did you achieve them?
Yes / No

5. If not, what can you do differently next time in order to secure a positive outcome?

PERSONAL RECORDS

LIFT/EXERCISE: DATE:

LIFT/EXERCISE: DATE:

LIFT/EXERCISE: DATE:

LIFT/EXERCISE: DATE:

LIFT/EXERCISE: DATE:

PERSONAL RECORDS

LIFT/EXERCISE: DATE:

LIFT/EXERCISE: DATE:

LIFT/EXERCISE: DATE:

LIFT/EXERCISE: DATE:

LIFT/EXERCISE: DATE:

NOTES AND RAMBLINGS / THINGS I NEED TO SAY TO MYSELF

If we expect to fail, we will fail.
We become what we think.
So expect to achieve, darling.

Made in the USA
Lexington, KY
01 September 2016